YOUR KNOWLEDGE HAS VALUE

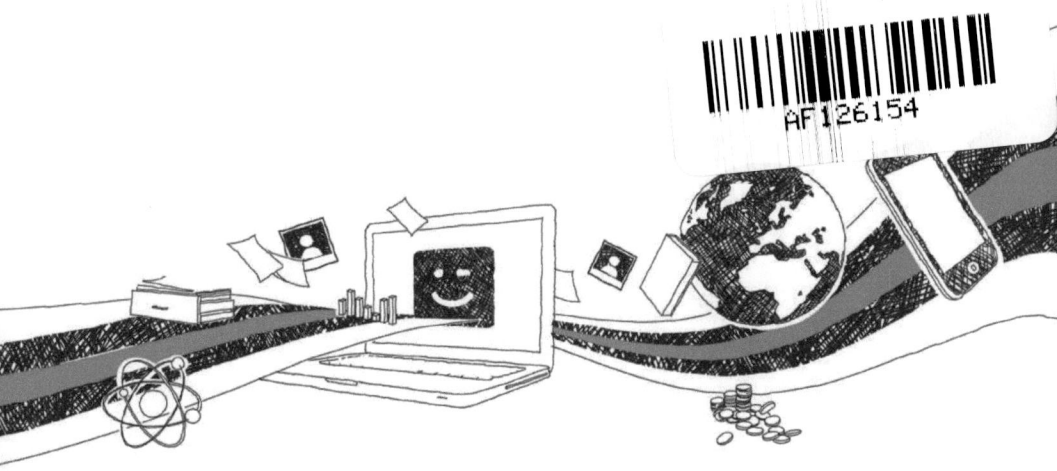

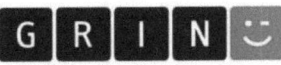

The Fatigue Management Program for Airport Workers in New Zealand. An Evaluation

Damien Hiquet

Bibliographic information published by the German National Library:

The German National Library lists this publication in the National Bibliography; detailed bibliographic data are available on the Internet at http://dnb.dnb.de.

ISBN: 9783346547514
This book is also available as an ebook.

© GRIN Publishing GmbH
Nymphenburger Straße 86
80636 München

Print and binding: Books on Demand GmbH, Norderstedt, Germany
Printed on acid-free paper from responsible sources.

The present work has been carefully prepared. Nevertheless, authors and publishers do not incur liability for the correctness of information, notes, links and advice as well as any printing errors.

GRIN web shop: https://www.grin.com/document/1151307

Evaluation of a Fatigue management programme for Airport workers

Damien Hiquet

2021

Table of contents

1. Executive summary

Airports, like hospitals, never close and, as such, healthcare providers and aviation professionals operate under a distinctive but shared set of circumstances (Feiner, 2017).

As a result, long and intensive shifts are common, sleep deprivation and fatigue are widespread.

Therefore, fatigue can be defined as the decreased capability to perform mental or physical work, produced as a function of inadequate sleep, circadian disruption, or time on task (Brown, 1994 as cited in Safety Institute of Australia, 2012).

Circadian disruption refers to wake and sleep that occur outside of the body's circadian rhythm. Circadian rhythms regulate different functions of the body to an average 24.2-hour cycle (Czeisler et al., 1999 as cited in Safety Institute of Australia, 2012). These rhythms are evident in functions such as sleep propensity (the ability to initiate and maintain sleep), body temperature, performance and mood (S. S. Campbell & Murphy, 2007; Clark, Watson, & Leeka, 1989; Kryger, Roth, & Carskadon, 1994; Lack & Lushington, 2003 as cited in Safety Institute of Australia, 2012).

In "figure 1", the circadian rhythm of sleep propensity is shown and demonstrates how the homeostatic drive for sleep and the circadian system interact to regulate the sleep/wake cycle.

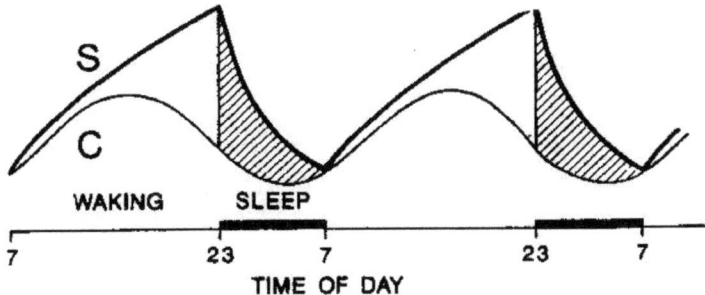

Figure 1: Borbély's model of sleep-wake regulation. Process S represents the homeostatic built-up of sleep pressure. Process C represents the circadian rhythm. When the distance between process S and process C is largest, sleep propensity will be highest (Borbély & Achermann, 1999 as cited in Moens, 2010).

The circadian rhythm has peaks and troughs. The circadian nadir – the low point of the circadian rhythm which typically occurs in the early hours of the morning also called the window of circadian low (WOCL).

During this time, core body temperature is at its lowest and sleep propensity is at its highest (Dijk & Czeisler, 1995 as cited in Safety Institute of Australia, 2012). Sleep during the circadian nadir is associated with greater restorative value and feelings of rest upon waking (Åkerstedt, Hume, Minors, & Waterhouse, 1997 as cited in Safety Institute of Australia, 2012).

If wake occurs during this time, the individual is likely to experience a depressed mood and is unlikely to perform at an optimum level (Åkerstedt, 2003; Frey, Badia, & Wright, 2004; T. H. Monk et al., 1997 as cited in Safety Institute of Australia, 2012).

In the hours following the circadian nadir, there is an increase in core body temperature and a decrease in sleep propensity, leading to waking. The peak of the circadian rhythm is when core body temperature is highest and sleep propensity is lowest, and typically occurs at approximately 17:00. This time of day is associated with high levels of function and alertness. Sleep occurring during the peak is likely to be restless and truncated (Åkerstedt, 2003 as cited in Safety Institute of Australia, 2012).

In summary, wake that occurs out of synchrony with the circadian drive for wakefulness is characterised by impaired functioning, excessive sleepiness and increased fatigue.

Also, sleep that occurs out of synchrony with the circadian rhythm is likely to be of reduced restorative value. Both of these circumstances are likely to result in increased fatigue ("figure 2").

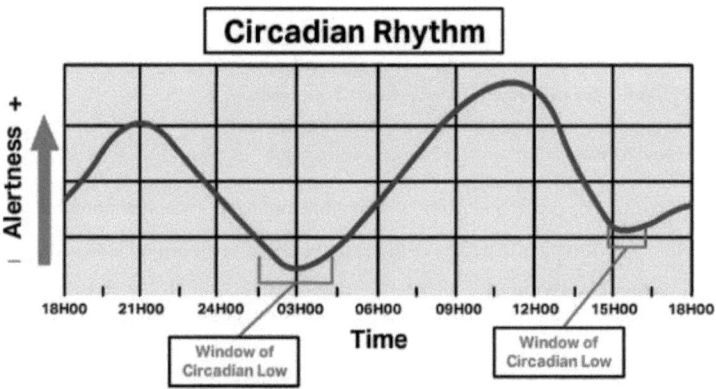

Figure 2: Window of circadian low (WOCL). Points daily minimum body temperature; more sleepy and least able to perform mental/physical tasks (IATA Training, 2021).

Besides, fatigue should be treated as an impairment, similar to being under the influence of alcohol or drugs as demonstrated by Dawson and Reid (1997) in "figure 3".

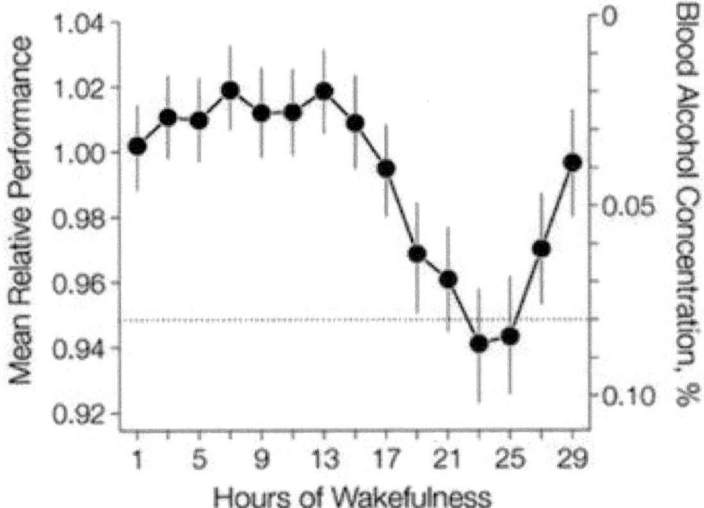

Figure 3: Performance in the sustained wakefulness condition expressed as mean relative performance and the percentage blood alcohol concentration equivalent (Dawson & Reid, 1997).

Thus, comparing means relative performance and blood alcohol concentration equivalent against hours of wakefulness clearly indicate that the effects of moderate sleep loss on performance are similar to moderate alcohol intoxication.

For instance, after seventeen hours of sustained wakefulness cognitive psychomotor performance decreased to a level equivalent to the performance impairment observed at a blood alcohol concentration of 0.05%. This is the proscribed level of alcohol intoxication in many western industrialised countries.

However, the authors believe that the performance impairment associated with shift work could be even greater than reported in their study.

Indeed, as about fifty per cent of shift workers do not sleep on the day before the first night shift, levels of fatigue on subsequent night shifts can be even higher (Dawson & Reid, 1997).

In "figure 4", Folkard and Tucker (2003) show the correlation between incidents/accidents and morning, afternoon and night shift with the last one having the biggest increase in the risk of incidents/accidents.

Simultaneously, they indicate what is the performance efficiency at a different time of the day. As shown, it has a negative value from midnight until six in the morning (Folkard & Tucker, 2003 as cited in Gregory, 2020).

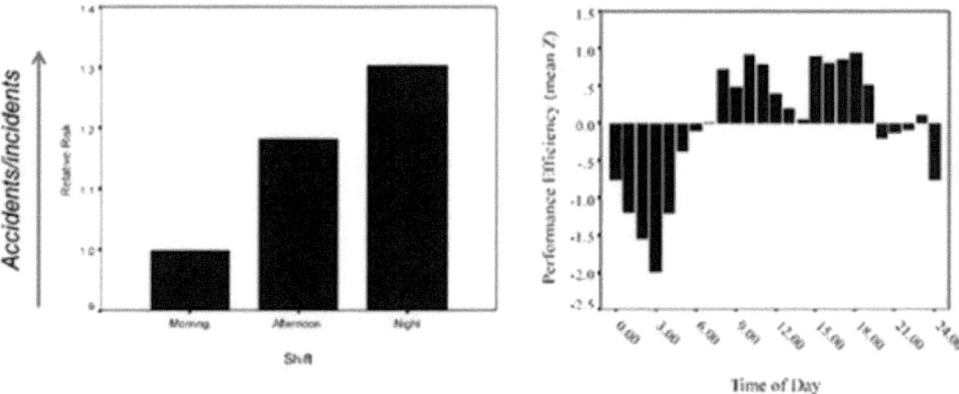

Figure 4: Industrial performance efficiency over the twenty-four hours/day
(Folkard & Tucker, 2003)

Furthermore, the authors prove that there is an increase of relative risk during the length of consecutive shifts. However, they are greater during successive night shifts ("Figure 5").

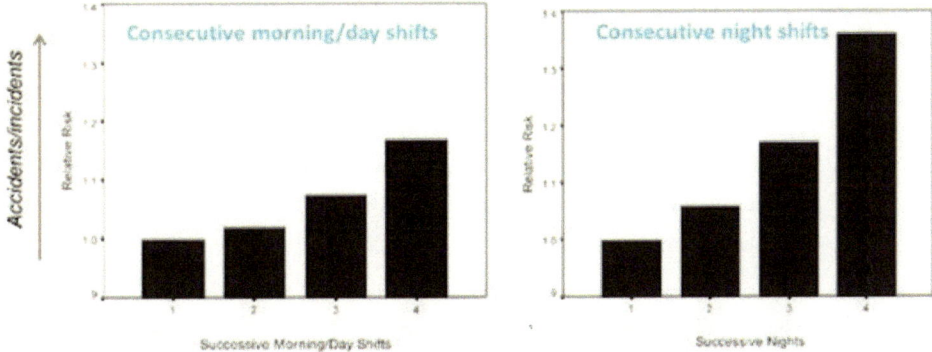

Figure 5: Consecutive work periods (Folkard & Tucker, 2003 as cited in Gregory, 2020)

In New Zealand, the Ministry of Transport has published on its website a graph measuring the percentage de crash where driver fatigue was a contributing factor, against the time of the day between 2017-2019 ("Figure 6").

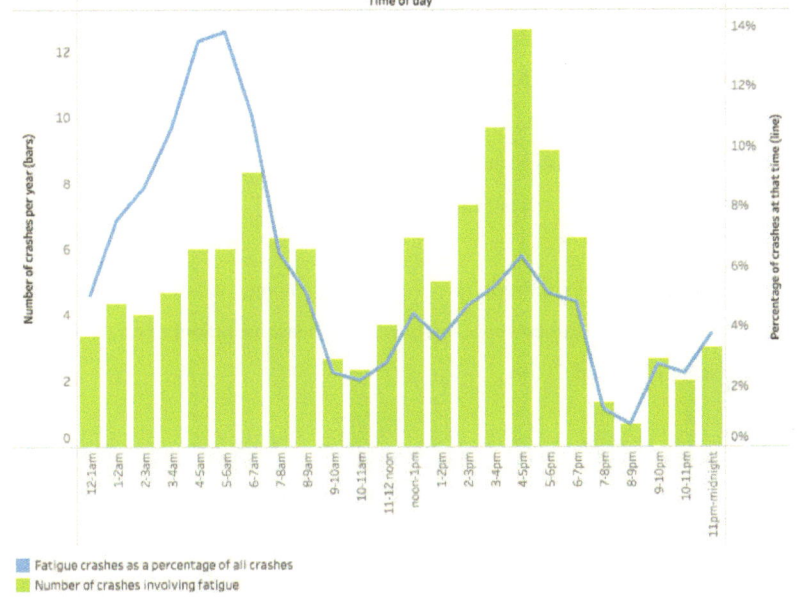

Fatigue crashes as a percentage of all crashes
Number of crashes involving fatigue

Figure 6: Fatal and serious injury crashes with driver fatigue as a contributing factor by time of day (annual average 2017 - 2019) (Ministry of Transport, 2020). (The figure is displayed larger on the last page.)

As shown, there are broad peaks in fatigue-related and serious, injury crashes in the early morning and through the afternoon.

Amongst the people to experience more likely fatigue while driving is the shift workers (Waka Kotahi NZ Transport Agency, 2021).

With the government Road to Zero strategy, stakeholders have also noted that factors such as long working hours can also impact the safety of workers travelling to and from their workplace (Pennington, 2020).

In her research, Dr Lilley of Otago University underscores that road crashes are by far the single largest cause of work-related deaths. She concludes that: "there's definitely a blind spot around organisational aspects such as risk management or safety culture ... or fatigue impairing performance, these often are not investigated in any great depth" (Lilley et al., 2019).

For instance, Maritime New Zealand has surveyed in January 2018 professional fishermen. More than half of the respondents (52%) has experienced mood swings as a result of fatigue, with even more (56%) admitting they would make mistakes on the job when fatigued. Then some fell asleep at the wheel (34%), made a bad decision (42%), and were easily distracted or unable to concentrate (39%).

Almost forty per cent claim to not have received any training on how to combat fatigue. This is despite having learned about safety either at maritime school or on the job (Maritime New Zealand, 2018).

According to IATA, fatigue as a human factor plays a significant role in thirty per cent of commercial aviation accidents (International Aviation Transport Association, 2021).

2. Purpose and objectives

Fatigue is an unavoidable consequence of modern airline operations due to shift work and crew duties which invariably are associated with some sleep disruption. There is a large variation between individuals in their ability to cope with sleep disruption and jet lag.

In section sixteen, the Health and Safety Work Act 2015 (HSWA) recognises fatigue as a hazard implying that the Person Conducting a Business or Undertaking (PCBU)must manage it.

For the civil aviation system, the International Civil Aviation Organisation (ICAO) has set the fundamental standards for fatigue risk management (FRM).

Nationally, the Civil Aviation Authority (CAA) is the workplace health and safety regulator under HSWA.

In general, the CAA administers the provisions of the HSWA for the aviation sector, with its jurisdiction covering:
- Work to prepare an aircraft for imminent flight;
- Work onboard an aircraft for imminent flight or while in operation; and
- Aircraft as workplaces while in operation.

Then, WorkSafe administers HSWA in respect of the aviation sector in all other circumstances (Civil Aviation Authority, 2021).

As an adherent of the ACC Accredited Employer Programme (AEP), the organisation must comply with the components of the scheme (Accident Corporation Compensation, 2017,).

Therefore, managing fatigue has a high priority for the organisation and forms part of the Safety Management System (SMS) as it is considered a critical risk.

However, ICAO requires the airline to distinguish Fatigue Risk Management System (FRMS) policy from the general SMS policy(International Aviation Transport Association, 2021).

Within the organisation, the FRMS must be distributed and reviewed periodically ("Figure 7").

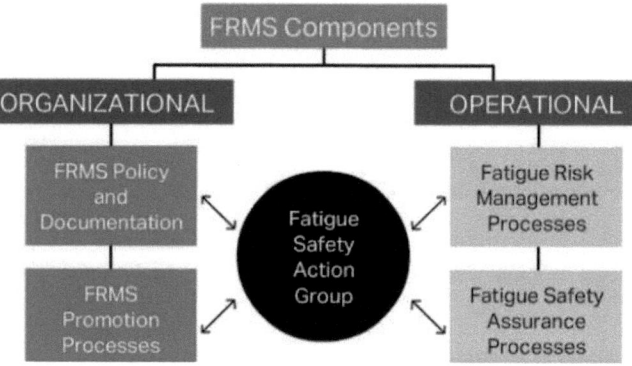

Figure 7: Fatigue Risk Management System (IATA, 2021).

Training programmes are part of the FRM promotion process.

Because the nature of airline operations is unique from many other occupations, fatigue can be mitigated with several evidence-based strategies. There are no "one-size fits all" approach to fatigue management and no single strategy will fully eliminate the threat of fatigue in the workplace. Numerous individual-level, environmental factors, social factors, scheduling and work-related factors, as well as many other known or latent factors must be considered when developing an FRMS. What works for aircrew may not work for ground staff (Patterson et al., 2015).

Thus, the participants are diverse, and the FRMS training programmes must be adapted to suit the needs of each group (e.g., crewmembers, operational decision-makers, the person who design, rosters and schedules).

Also, it includes senior management, particularly the executive accountable for the FRMS and senior leadership in any department managing operations within the FRMS.

Nevertheless, all groups require basic education about scientific principles. That includes dynamics of sleep loss and recovery, the effects of the daily cycle of the circadian body clock, the influence of workload, how these factors interact with operational demand to produce fatigue, and information on how to manage their fatigue and sleep issues.

Indeed, it is useful for all groups to know the causes and consequences of fatigue in their operations and the importance of accurate data.

Additionally, it promotes shared responsibility and the worker to identify fatigue in itself and others.

Following the ICAO recommendation, the organisation combine fatigue training with other training programmes (e.g., crew resource management, SMS). This way it makes things interesting for the learners (ICAO, 2018).

However, the decision to combine training programmes also depends on the four ways of the delivery method used:
• Live class training with a qualified instructor
• Computed-based training (CBT)
• E-learning is a web-based training
• Fatigue manual, which involves self-study with an assessment

3. Evaluation process

Chronic sleep restriction below seven hours per night is associated with significant daytime cognitive dysfunction that accumulated to levels comparable to that found after severe acute total sleep deprivation.

For instance, aviation maintenance technicians (AMT) have been working long hours to compensate for the wage reductions since the 9/11 terrorist attacks.

In 2001 before the attack, a study examining AMT sleep and rest periods revealed AMTs were only getting about five hours of sleep, on average, per night (Johnson, Mason, Hall, & Watson, 2013 cited in Banks et al., 2013, p.1).

Therefore, developing fatigue countermeasures training tailored to AMT is an obvious starting place and an evaluation is conducted on the initial delivery of the training in a classroom setting.

In "figure 8", the training outline covered three main topics: sleep basics, fatigue basics, and fatigue countermeasures.

Sleep Basics	Fatigue Basics	Fatigue Countermeasures
Sleep Process	Fatigue Hazards	Work Breaks
Circadian Rhythm	Causes of Fatigue	Napping
Sleep Disorders	How to Assess Fatigue	Sleep Routine
Sleep Debt	Fatigue Symptoms	Sleeping Environment

Figure 8: Content covered in the training

Training objectives were: (a) remember symptoms of fatigue and fatigue countermeasures, (b) recognise the importance of managing fatigue risk, and (c) incorporate practical recommendations for fatigue prevention and management into a daily routine. Training outcome measures used to determine if the objectives were met included: gains in knowledge, increased awareness of fatigue risk and the importance of managing fatigue, and an increase in self-report of fatigue-related positive behaviours and reduction of negative behaviours at home and work.

Following the Kirkpatrick model, the delivered training was evaluated on four levels: learning (positive change in knowledge of and attitude toward countering fatigue), behaviour modification (change in fatigue management behaviours at home and work), transfer (application of what was taught at home and work), and reaction to the training experience.

For the methodology of the evaluation, a pretest-posttest design with a follow-up assessment was used to evaluate the training.

Before conducting statistical comparisons of the evaluation data, developing an instrument simple and reliable for assessing fatigue is necessary (Horisberger et al., 2019).

However, fatigue is difficult to evaluate and standardise. In "figure 9", the Fatigue Assessment Scale (FAS) is a simple ten-item self-reported with response values (five-point scale) summed to produce a total score questionnaire designed to assess fatigue (Michielsen et al, 2003 cited in Horisberger et al., 2019).

The following 10 statements refer to how you usually feel. For each statement you can choose one out of five answer categories, varying from *never* to *always*. 1 = *never*; 2 = *sometimes*; 3 = *regularly*; 4 = *often*; 5 = *always*.

	Never	Sometimes	Regularly	Often	Always
1. I am bothered by fatigue (WHOQOL)	1	2	3	4	5
2. I get tired very quickly (CIS)	1	2	3	4	5
3. I don't do much during the day (CIS)	1	2	3	4	5
4. I have enough energy for everyday life (WHOQOL)	1	2	3	4	5
5. Physically, I feel exhausted (CIS)	1	2	3	4	5
6. I have problems starting things (FS)	1	2	3	4	5
7. I have problems thinking clearly (FS)	1	2	3	4	5
8. I feel no desire to do anything (CIS)	1	2	3	4	5
9. Mentally, I feel exhausted	1	2	3	4	5
10. When I am doing something, I can concentrate quite well (CIS)	1	2	3	4	5

Reprinted from Michielsen et al. [1]. Copyright © 2003, with permission from Elsevier.
Note: The abbreviations after the items indicate the scale from which the items has been abstracted. The following are the scales:
CIS - Checklist Individual Strength
WHOQOL - World Health Organization Quality of Life assessment instrument
FS - Fatigue Scale

Figure 9: Fatigue Assessment Scale (Shahid et al., 2012).

4. Conclusions and results

In the United States, fatigue countermeasures training has been used for more than two decades across industries (railroad, trucking, and water transport) with 24/7 operations, to mitigate on-the-job fatigue risks (Nicholson & Stone, 1987 as cited in Banks et al., 2013, p. 1). The training can be beneficial to both the individual and the organisation. Individuals who replace bad sleep and health habits with good ones benefit from improved sleep quality and quantity, while the organisation benefits from improvements in performance and fewer safety-reducing turnovers, absenteeism, and moral issues (Kerin & Aguirre, 2005 as cited in Banks et al., 2013).

4.1 Learning

There was an immediate impact of training on attendee fatigue-related knowledge. Average test scores increased by fifty per cent going from fifty per cent correct before training to 75 .2% correct at the end of training ("Figure 10").

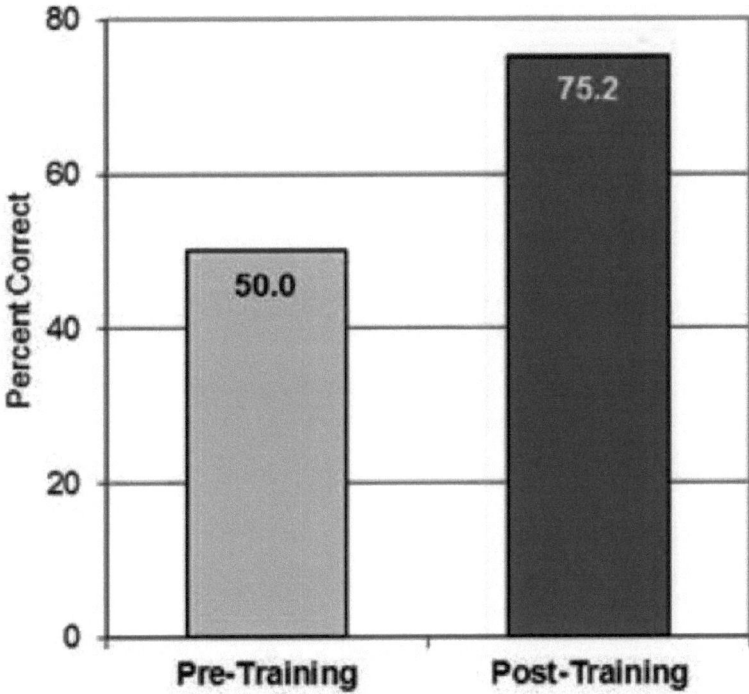

Figure 10: Immediate impact of training on knowledge test scores (Banks et al., 2013, p.4)

4.2 Behavior modification

Shifts in attendee awareness of the importance of managing fatigue and self-efficacy trended in the positive direction, training only had an immediate positive impact on awareness of the importance of not being fatigued at work.

Indeed, "Figure 11" shows the positive shift in awareness of importance and commitment to managing fatigue realised immediately after training did not persist six weeks later.

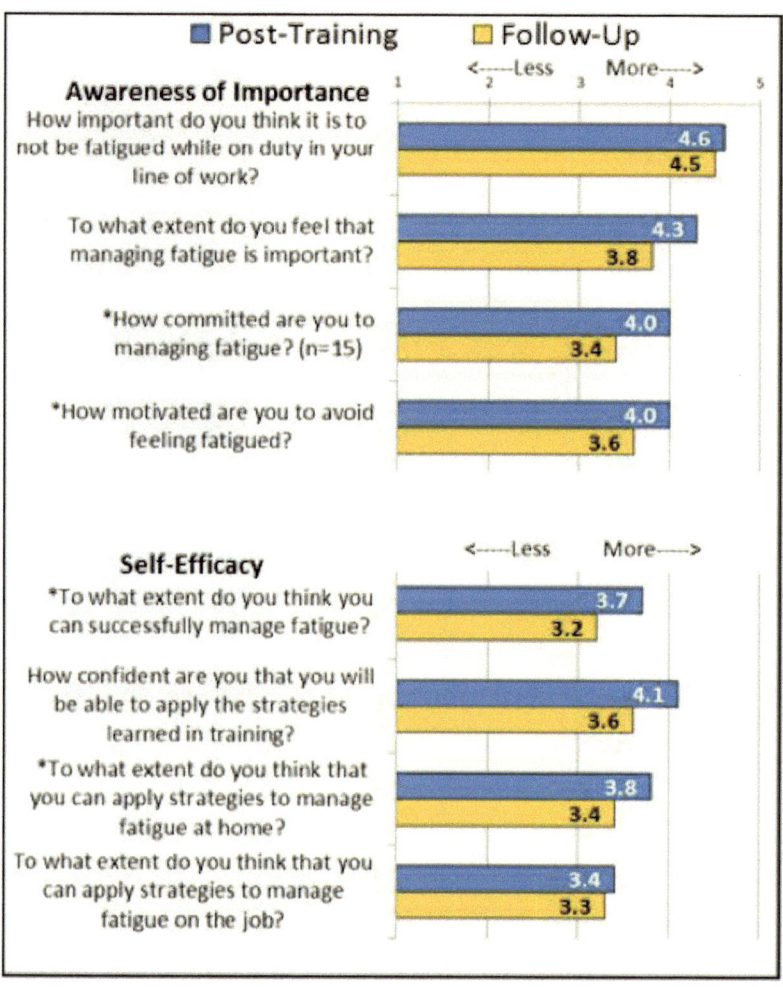

Figure 11: Retention of attitudes between training and follow-up ((Banks et al., 2013, p. 6)

4.3 Transfer

In "Figure 12", transfer refers to the use of fatigue countermeasures covered in training in the home and work environments implying that the environments offer support for and opportunities to employ countermeasure recommendations.

Thus, this is more likely the case at home, where there is more individual control than at work.

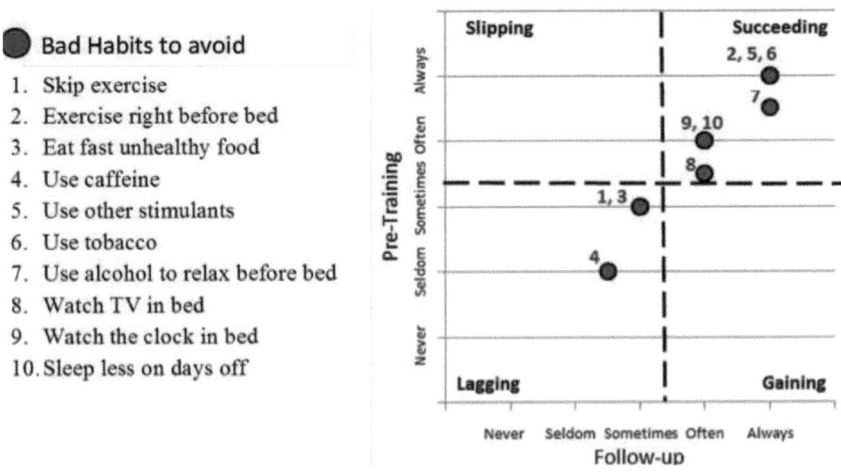

Figure 12: Avoidance of bad habits before training versus follow-up (Banks et al., 2013, p. 9)

4.4 Reaction to the training experience

Instructional qualities are assessed on a five-point Likert scale, with the following labels: Strongly Disagree, Disagree, Neutral, Agree, and Strongly Agree.

For instance, results based on AMT attendees who provided data on their reaction to the training experience were overwhelmingly positive. All attendees agreed that the training was informative and useful. The vast majority agreed that training was interesting, worthwhile, and should be conducted for others (97%) and that the material was well organised (96%) and presented at the appropriate level (94%) (Banks et al., 2013, p. 13).

4.5 Conclusion

The positive shift is notable given the resistance of attitudes and behaviours to change (Erber, Hodges, & Wilson, 1995 as cited in Banks et al., 2013, p. 13).

 Therefore, observed improvements were in awareness of the importance of not being fatigued at work and commitment to manage fatigue increased immediately after training

Then, modifications of sleep routines reported at follow-up (more likely to sleep in the bedroom and block out noise from the bedroom at follow-up).

However, few reported changes in work behaviours at follow-up and a rebound occurred back to pre-training levels in employees commitment, motivation, and self-efficacy toward managing fatigue.

5. Recommendations

The effectiveness of the training is partly attributable to the customisation of content for the targeted personnel (e.g., AMT, crew, airports) and the personalisation of fatigue health risks and benefits of fatigue management.

When resistance exists, modifying and sustaining new behaviours and attitudes toward fatigue can be challenging, since lifestyle changes are required.

However, the organisation can also productively engage resistance when developing or revising policies and procedures to reduce fatigue-related safety risks by (Ford & Ford, 2010 as cited in Banks et al., 2013, p. 13):

- involving employees (e.g., health and safety representatives)
- focusing on the purpose of the change
- collecting data to develop evidence-based training
- integrating self-fatigue report for all employees report through its SMS
- resolving past issues
- clarifying objectives and strategies
- improving the implementation plan

Nevertheless, productive engagement from the organisation requires a commitment to reduce fatigue risk on the job (i.e., fatigue policy), otherwise, employees old patterns of behaviours will persist.

Likewise, the lack of engagement from the PCBU may contribute to employees feeling powerless to manage fatigue due to limited or poor control over the work environment, the work schedule, and the accelerated pace and elevated pressure to perform.

Because there are no regulatory look-back rest requirements unlike flying crew, airline shift workers appear to be susceptible to high levels of physical and cognitive fatigue.

Alike crews, shift workers perform consecutive extended shifts before returning home.

Therefore, the organisation FRMS should integrate all categories of workers impacted by fatigue and not only flying personnel.

Then, the risk posed by fatigue in the workplace may be managed, to an extent, in the same way, that many other hazards are managed in the workplace.

But, the implementation of FRMS requires an understanding of the science of fatigue and its evolution as a recognised hazard. The unique challenge associated with fatigue management lies in recognising that fatigue-management interventions have technical, social and cultural implications. Managing these implications in line with regulatory, organisational and individual requirements is imperative for the success of any fatigue risk management system. (Gander et al., 2011 as cited in Safety Institute of Australia, 2012).

Once the system is well developed, it becomes a shared responsibility between the PCBU and its well-trained worker which should continuously feedback its employer with fatigue reports in order to build data but also to improve training.

References

Accident Corporation Compensation. (2017). *Accredited Employers Programme*. https://
www.acc.co.nz/assets/business/acc440-aep-audit.pdf

Banks, J. O., Wenzel, B. M., Avers, K. E., & Hauck, E. L. (2013). *An evaluation of
aviation maintenance fatigue countermeasures training*. Federal Aviation
Administration. https://apps.dtic.mil/sti/pdfs/ADA603521.pdf

Civil Aviation Authority. (2021). *Fatigue risk management*. https://www.aviation.govt.nz/
safety/human-factors/fatigue-risk-management/

Dawson, D., & Reid, K. (1997, July 17). *Fatigue, alcohol and performance impairment*.
Nature. https://www.nature.com/articles/40775#citeas

Feiner, N. (2017). *Flying fatigue in twentieth-century Britain: An uncertain zone* [Doctoral
dissertation]. https://ore.exeter.ac.uk/repository/bitstream/handle/10871/31209/
FeinerN.pdf?sequence=1&isAllowed=y

Gregory, K. (2020, August 20). *Shiftwork & managing fatigue* [Video]. https://mediaex-
server.larc.nasa.gov/Academy/Play/70eee2f69f3243a5b97c92b199d25d8f1d

Horisberger, A., Courvoisier, D., & Ribi, C. (2019, March 25). *The fatigue assessment
scale as a simple and reliable tool in systemic lupus erythematosus: A cross-
sectional study*. Arthritis Research & Therapy. https://arthritis-
research.biomedcentral.com/articles/10.1186/s13075-019-1864-4

ICAO. (2018). *Doc 9859 Safety Management Manual*. SKYbrary Aviation Safety. https://
www.skybrary.aero/bookshelf/books/5863.pdf

International Aviation Transport Association. (2021, April 21). *Fatigue management fundamentals* [E-Learning]. IATA Training. https://www.iata.org/en/training/ courses/fatigue-mgt-fundamentals/tals72/en/ fbclid=IwAR1psUWTJAIlmCmhuO4ybhNJWxjUobnD77MPLsEpOk4v5iqXfKy_61ChU gU

Lilley, R., McNoe, B., Davie, G., Horsburgh, S., & Maclennan, B. (2019, May 6). *Identifying opportunities to prevent work-related fatal injury in New Zealand using 40 years of coronial records: Protocol for a retrospective case review study.* Injury Epidemiology. https://injepijournal.biomedcentral.com/articles/10.1186/ s40621-019-0193-z

Maritime New Zealand. (2018). *Fatigue in commercial fishing.* https:// www.maritimenz.govt.nz/commercial/safety/health-and-safety/fatigue/documents/ MNZ-Fatigue-research-2018.pdf

Ministry of Transport. (2020). *Safety — Annual statistics.* https://www.transport.govt.nz/ statistics-and-insights/safety-annual-statistics/sheet/fatigue

Moens, S. (2010, December 6). *Homeostatic and circadian processes underlying the sleep-wake cycle.* NeuroSomnia. https://smoens.wordpress.com/2010/12/06/homeostatic-and-circadian-processes-underlying-the-sleep-wake-cycle-1/

Parliamentary Counsel Office. (2015). *Health and Safety at Work Act 2015 no 70* (as at 01 December 2020), Public Act 16 interpretation – New Zealand legislation. https:// www.legislation.govt.nz/act/public/2015/0070/latest/DLM5976687.html? search=sw_096be8ed81a49df3_Fatigue_25_se&p=1&sr=0

Patterson, D., Weaver, M., & Guyette, F. X. (2015, July 28). *5 evidence-based countermeasures for EMS fatigue.* EMS1. https://www.ems1.com/ems-products/

furniture/articles/5-evidence-based-countermeasures-for-ems-fatigue-
zWehrGbhumjWqPxq/

Pennington, P. (2020, January 24). *Number of work-related deaths reported goes up.* RNZ.
https://www.rnz.co.nz/news/national/408058/number-of-work-related-deaths-
reported-goes-up

Safety Institute of Australia. (2012). *Psychosocial hazards: Fatigue.* The OHS Body of
Knowledge. https://www.ohsbok.org.au/wp-content/uploads/2019/07/20-
Fatigue-2012.pdf

Shahid, A., Wilkinson, K., & Marcu, S. (2012). *STOP, THAT and one hundred other sleep
scales.* Perelman School of Medicine | Perelman School of Medicine at the
University of Pennsylvania. https://www.med.upenn.edu/cbti/assets/user-content/
documents/Fatigue%20Assessment%20Scale%20(FAS).pdf

Waka Kotahi NZ Transport Agency. (2021). *Driver fatigue.* https://www.nzta.govt.nz/
safety/what-waka-kotahi-is-doing/education-initiatives/fatigue/

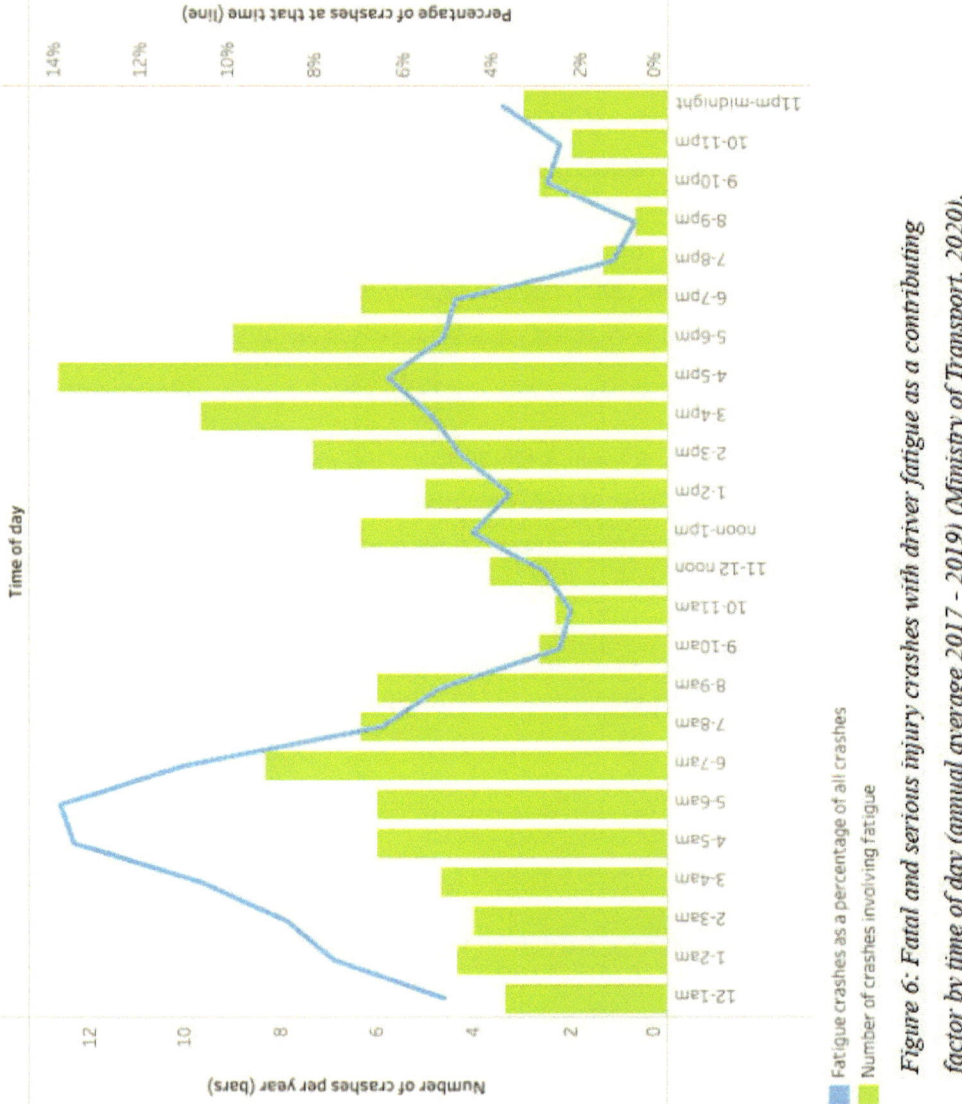

Figure 6: Fatal and serious injury crashes with driver fatigue as a contributing factor by time of day (annual average 2017 - 2019) (Ministry of Transport, 2020).

see p. 8